Hairstyles

Written by Kathryn Diane Grace

Illustrated by Aundrea D. Hernandez

YOUR BOOKS
SAN ANTONIO, TEXAS

Special thanks to my family—
James Jr., James III, Carrie, Carla, Kristina,
the Youngs, and the Graces,
for your love, support, and encouragement.
And
praise to my Father for His many blessings.

with all my love,
KDG

Published by YOUR BOOKS

YOUR BOOKS
P.O. Box 700872
San Antonio, Texas 78270-0872

Library of Congress Catalog Card Number: 98-91232

ISBN 0-9653414-2-9 (HARDCOVER)
ISBN 0-9653414-3-7 (PAPERBACK)

Printed in the United States of America
First Printing, March 1998

This book is dedicated to
all the young girls
that need to know

You are beautiful just as you are.

Stand tall,
hold your head up high,
and be proud.

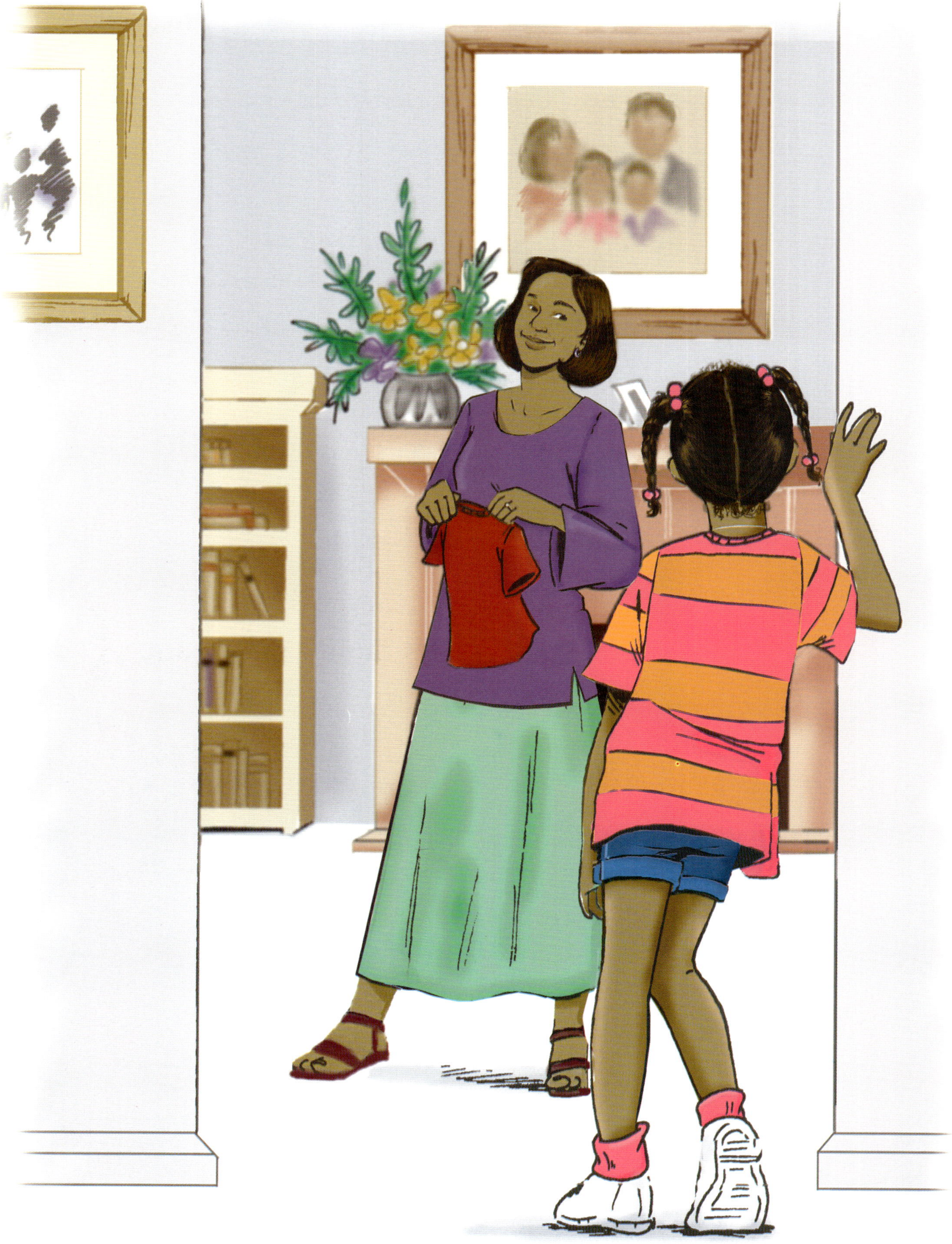

“Regina, bring me the comb and brush so I can do your hair,” her mother called from the family room Saturday morning.

“Mom, I don’t want you to do my hair,” Regina whined. She had just finished eating breakfast.

“Why not?” her mother asked.

Regina looked in the family room and said, “Sometimes it hurts my head.”

“Well, sweetheart, you may be a little tender-headed, but I have to comb out the tangles. It doesn’t hurt that bad. Our hair is strong and has a unique texture.”

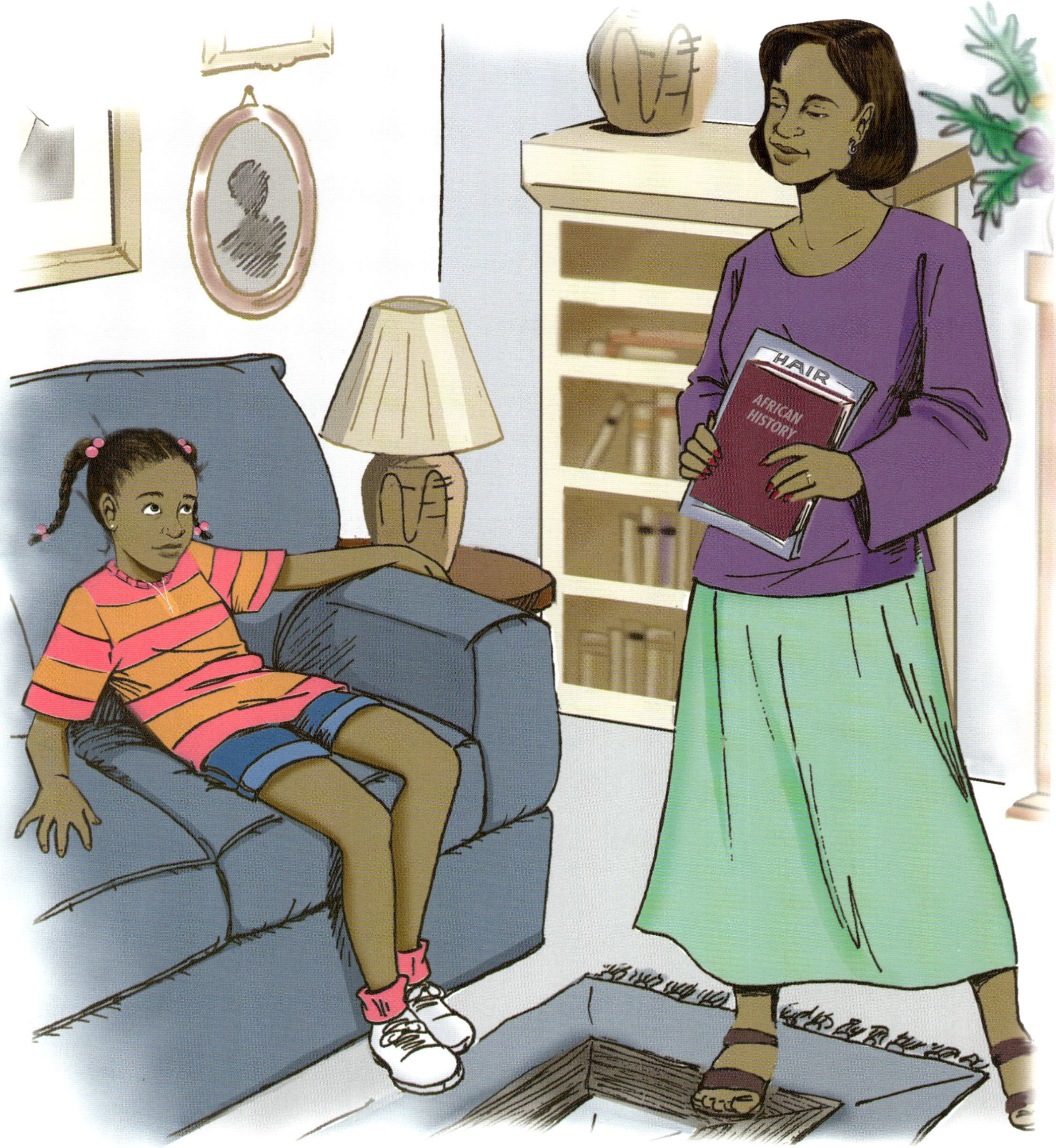
HAIR
AFRICAN HISTORY

“What does that mean?” Regina asked as she sat down.

“It means I can fix your hair in many different hairstyles.” Her mother walked over to the bookcase. “Did you know some of our hairstyles came from Africa? The styles were worn by African Queens and Princesses. I’ll show you my favorite picture.”

Regina’s mother selected a book and a magazine from the bookshelf. She walked to the couch and sat next to Regina. She placed the magazine on her lap and flipped through the book until she found the picture in the middle of the book.

“Mom, she looks beautiful!” Regina said, raising her eyebrows. “Was she an African Princess?”

“No, she was an African Queen.”

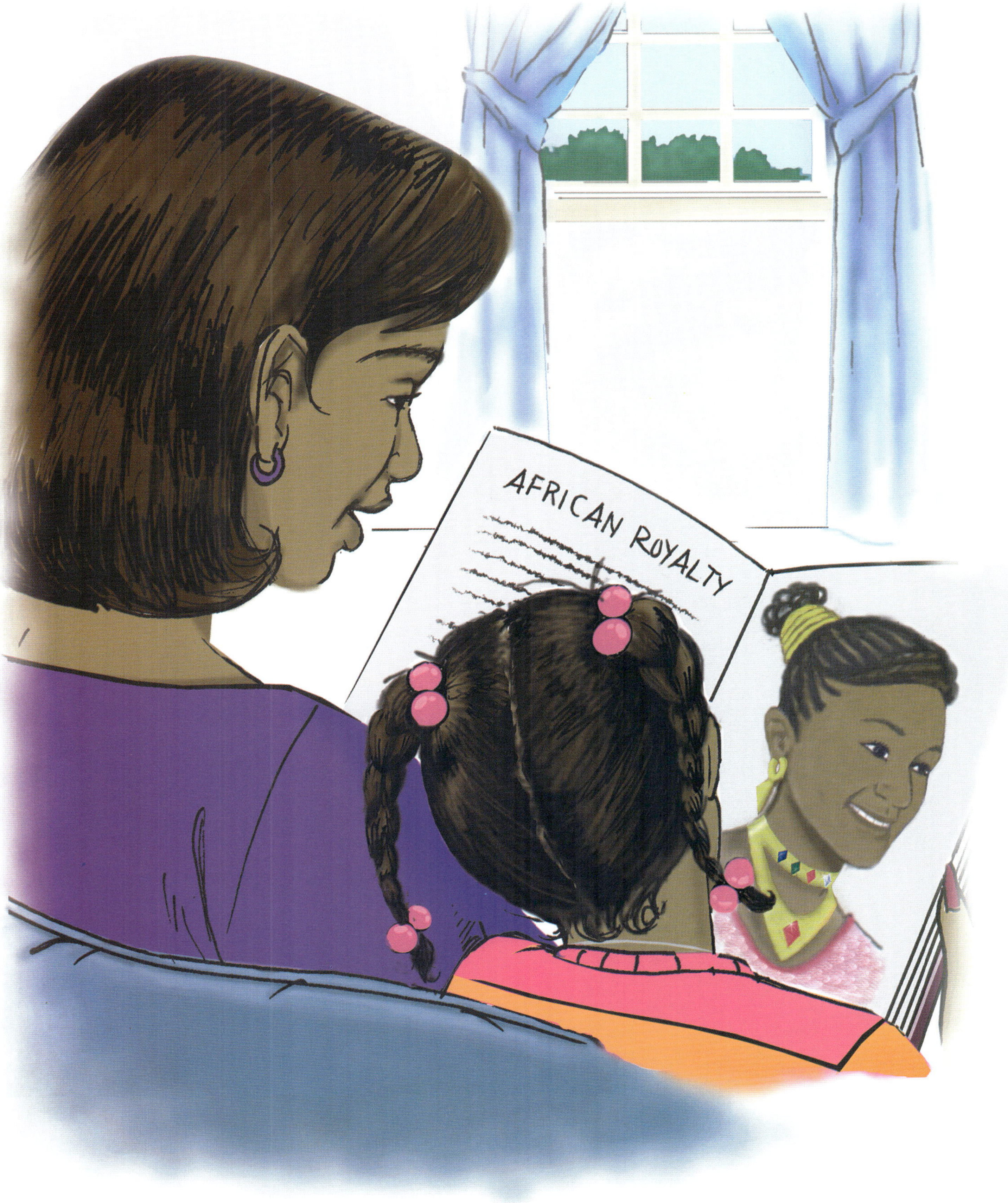
AFRICAN ROYALTY

They looked at several other pictures. Then her mother closed the book and placed it on the table. "I can arrange your hair in pretty hairstyles, too. How do you want me to fix your hair this morning?"

"I don't know," said Regina, grinning.

"I'll show you some pictures, and you try to imagine what the hairstyles would look like on you." Her mother opened the magazine. Regina turned the pages. It showed different hairstyles on each page.

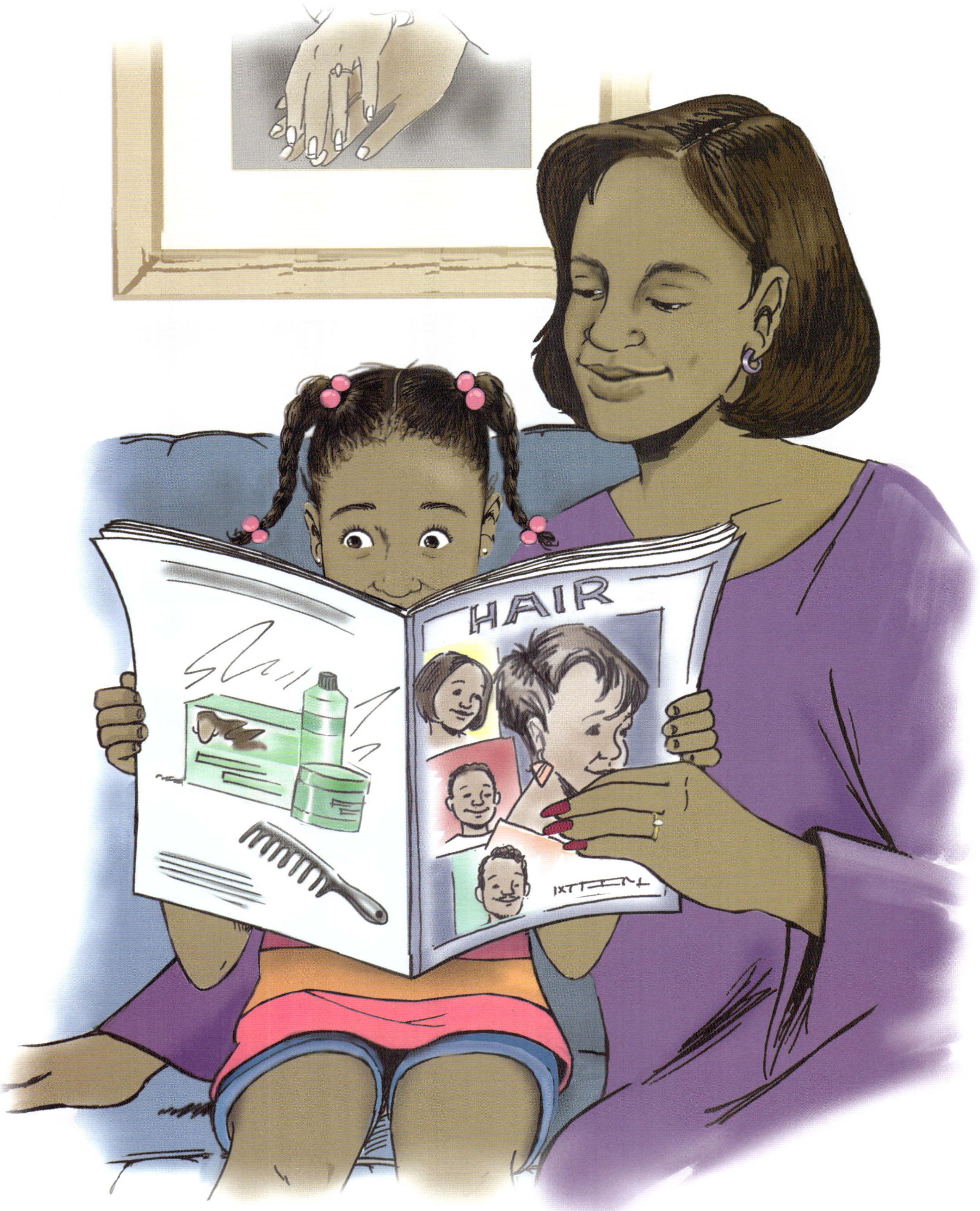
HAIR

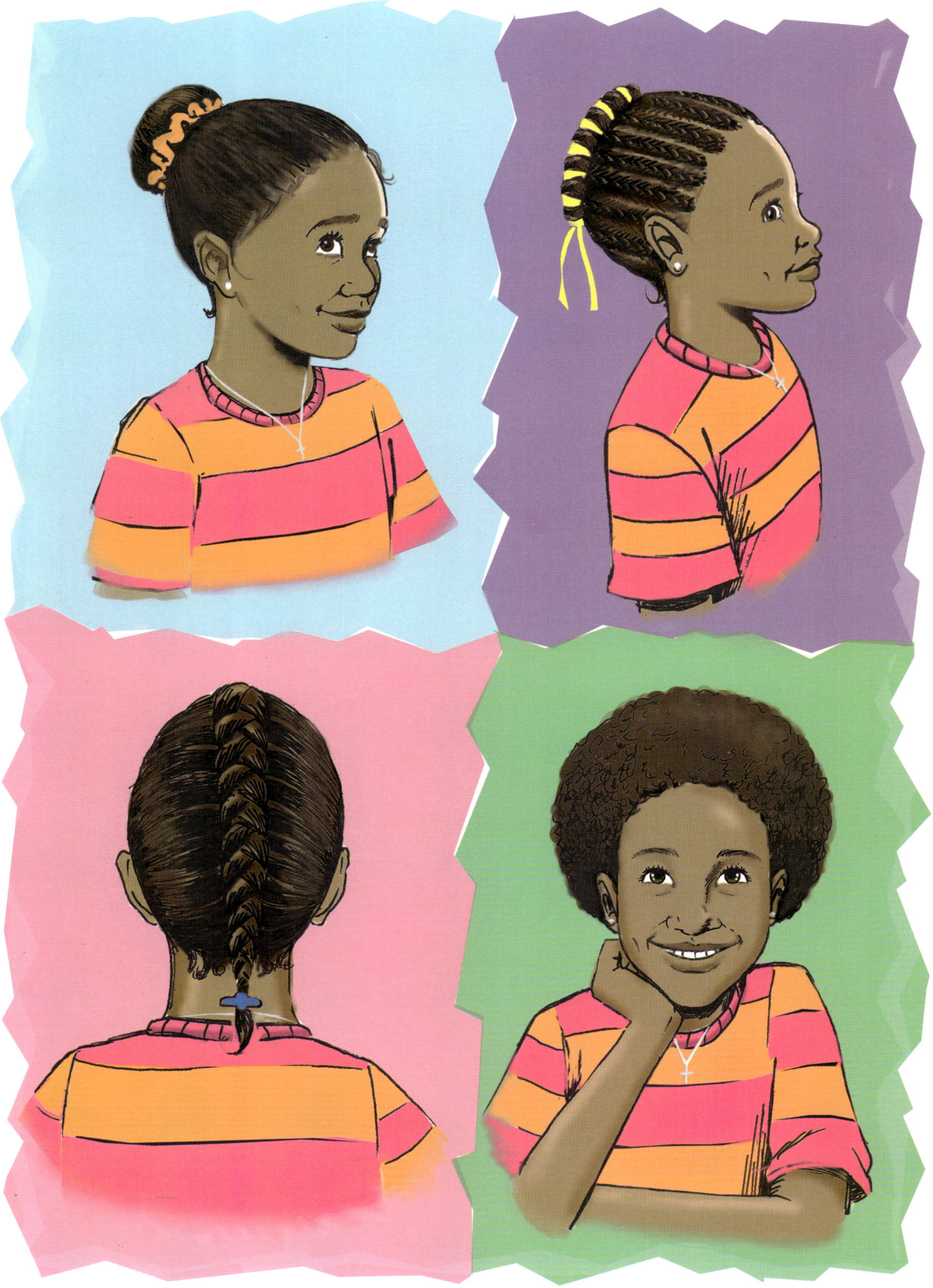

"Do you want your hair pulled back in a bun? Or do you want cornrows in a circle with ribbons wrapped around them?"

Regina smiled. She did not answer, so her mother continued to point at other pictures.

"Do you want one french braid? Or do you want your hair in an afro?"

Regina giggled shyly and shook her head.

“Would you like extensions?” Her mother paused. “Or do you want braids with ponytail holders and barrettes?”

Regina grinned and shrugged her shoulders.

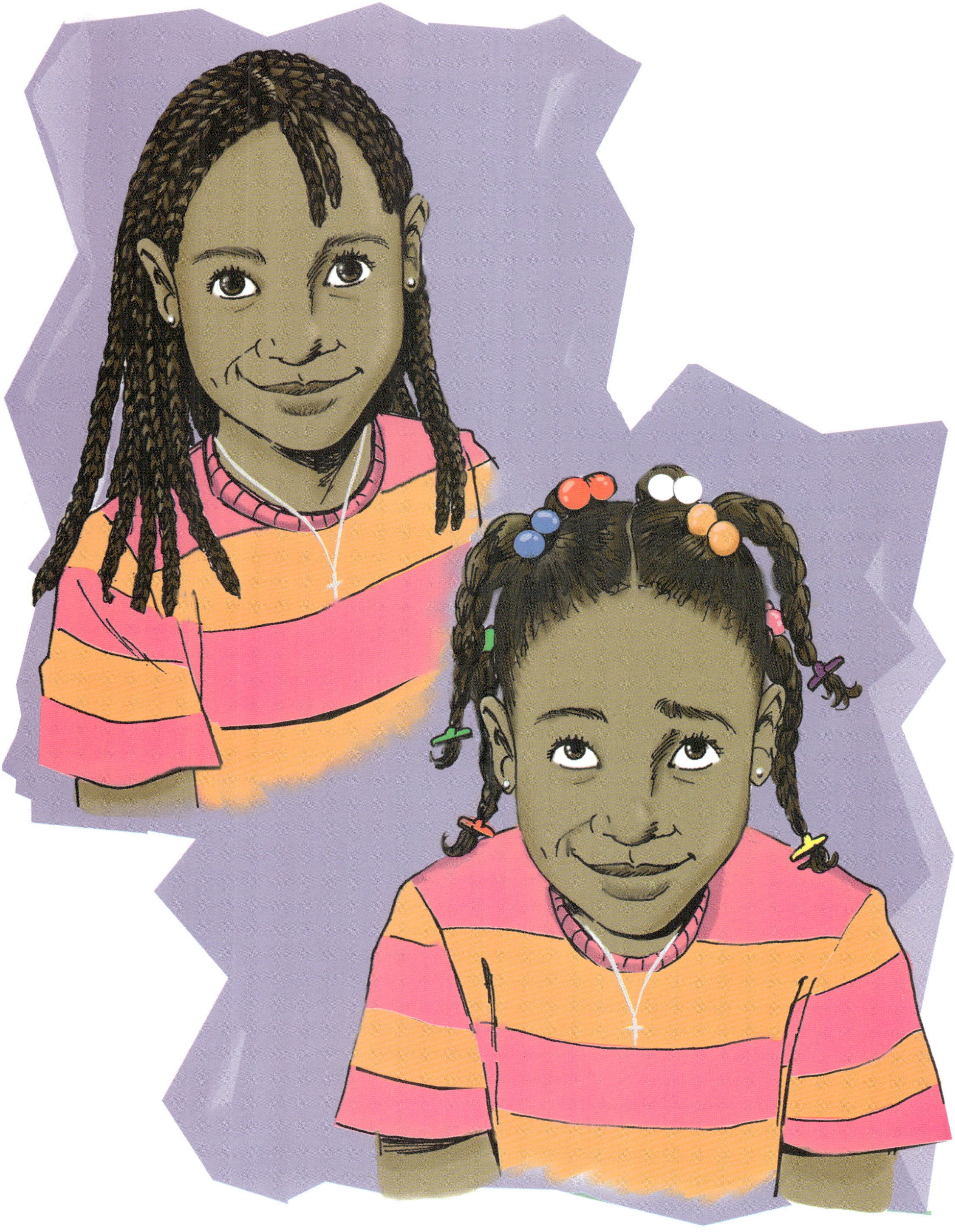

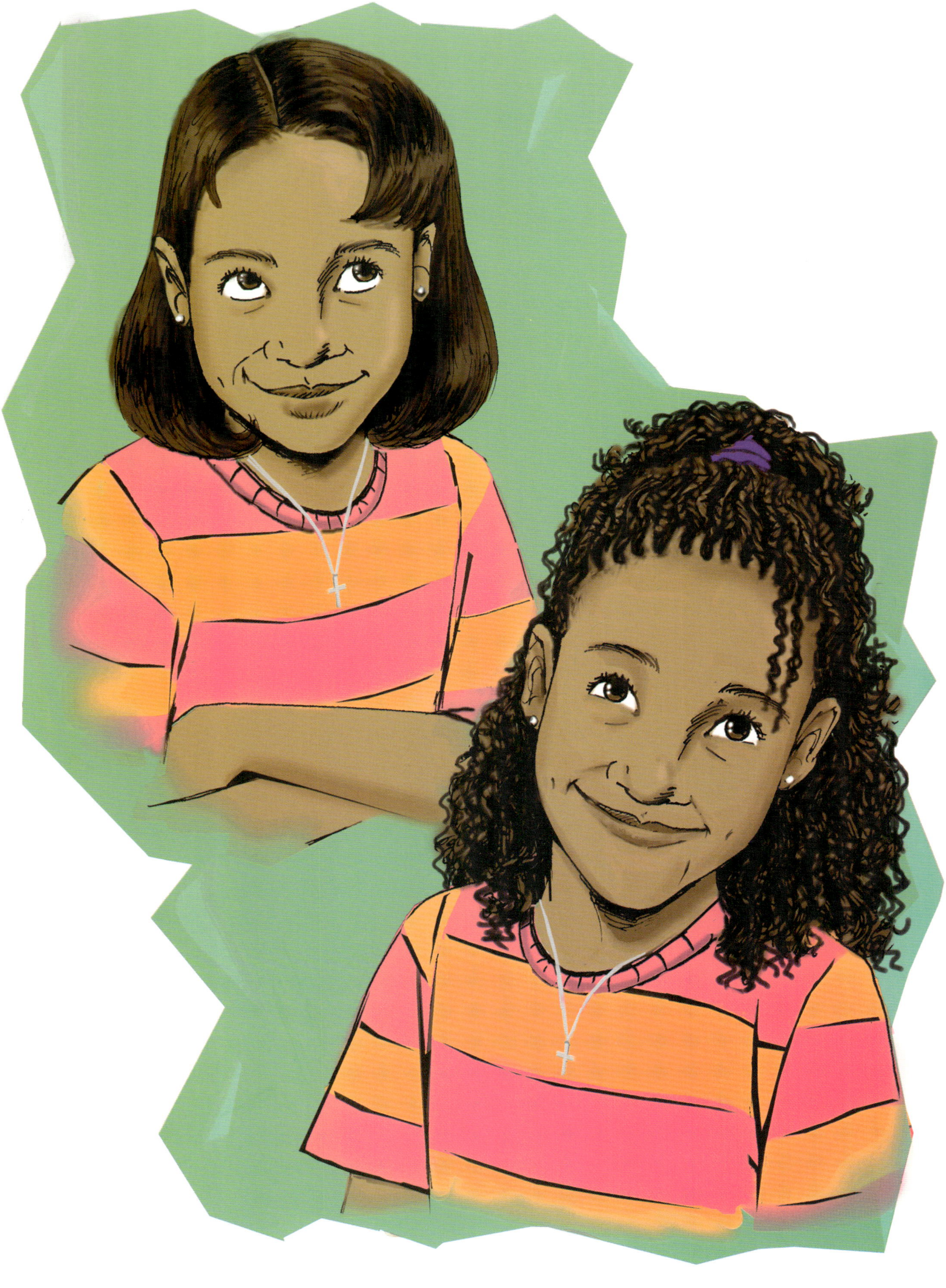

“Do you want your hair pressed with a straightening comb and curled at the ends?” her mother asked. “That’s almost like my hairstyle if you move the part to the other side. Do you like that?”

“Yeah, it’s nice.”

“No, it would make you look like a teenager,” her mother said as she pointed to another picture. “Oh, this style is cute. I think they call it crochet braids.”

After imagining the styles on her head, Regina turned the page.

“Do you want a ponytail with bangs?”

Her mother stopped and closed the magazine. “There are more hairstyles, but I’ll let you pick one of the styles I just showed you.”

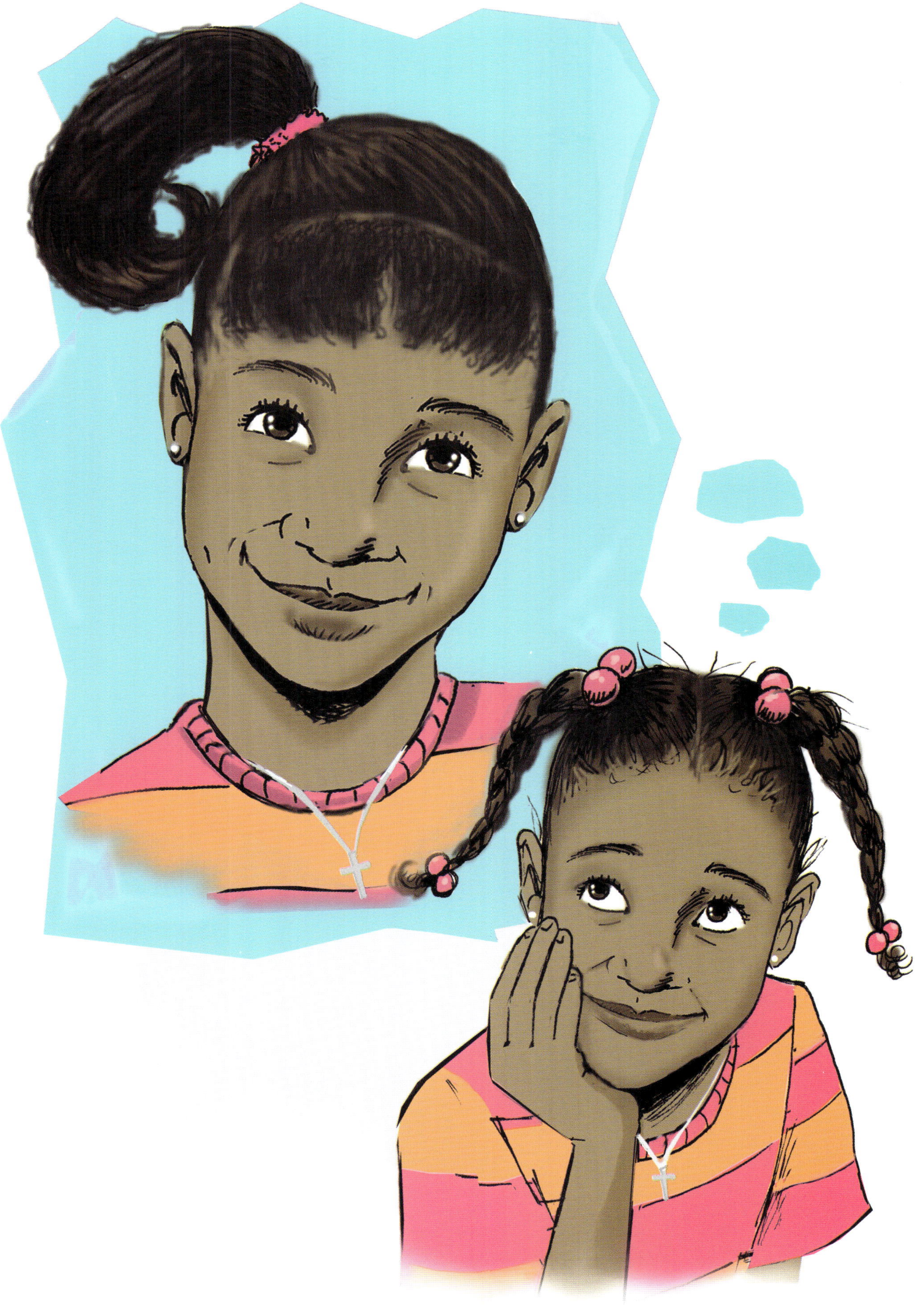

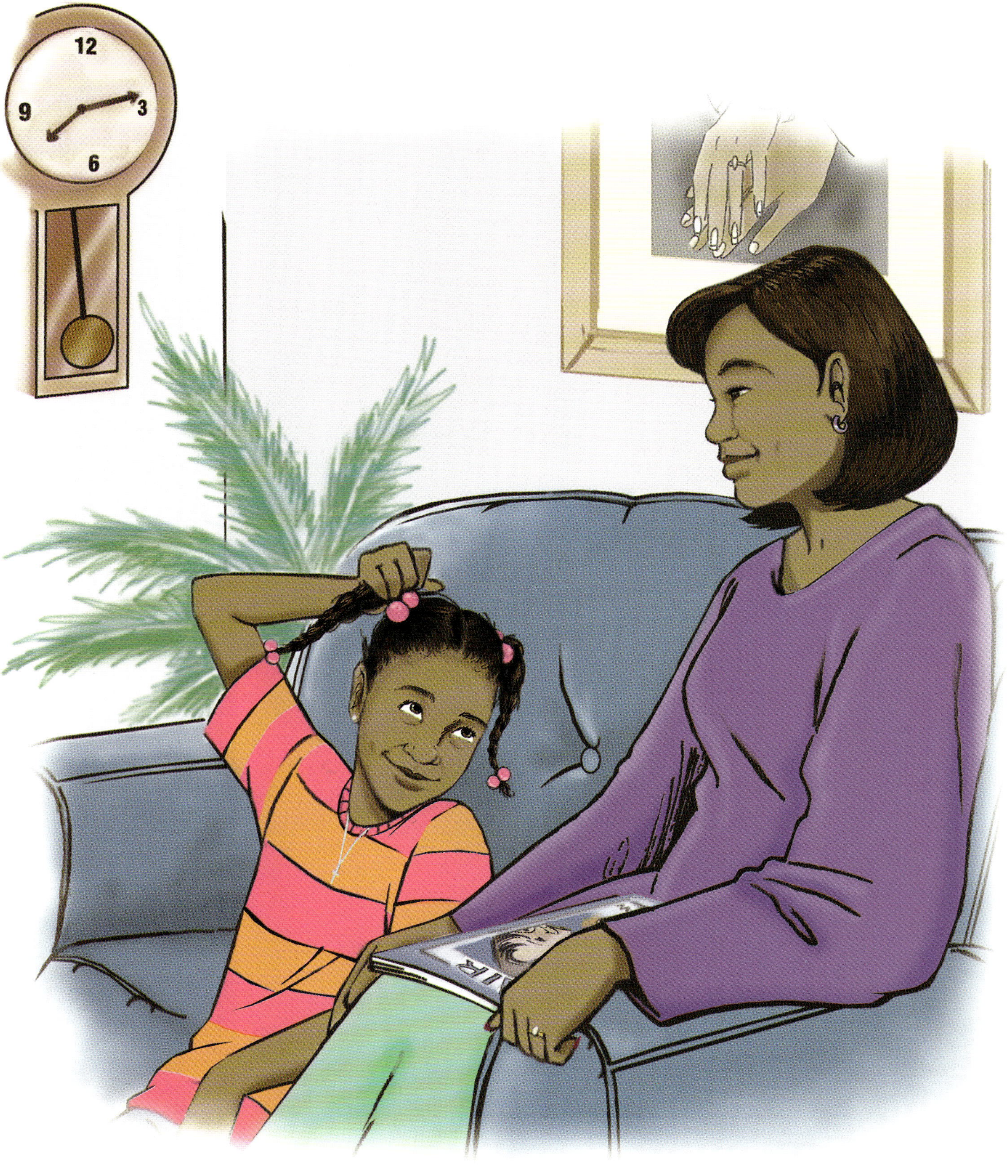
12
9
3
6

“Wow, all these great hairstyles for me! Mom, you can fix my hair a lot of different ways.” Regina reached up and felt her hair. “You’re right. It is strong.” She paused and said, “You can make cornrows today and a ponytail tomorrow.”

“If I make cornrows, I won’t have to take them out tomorrow,” her mother said. “They can stay in for weeks, as long as your hair looks neat. I can even wash your hair while it’s braided.”

“Okay, I’ll pick... uh... it’s so hard to choose.” Regina thought for a moment. All of a sudden, she had an idea. She whispered something in her mother’s ear. Her mother nodded.

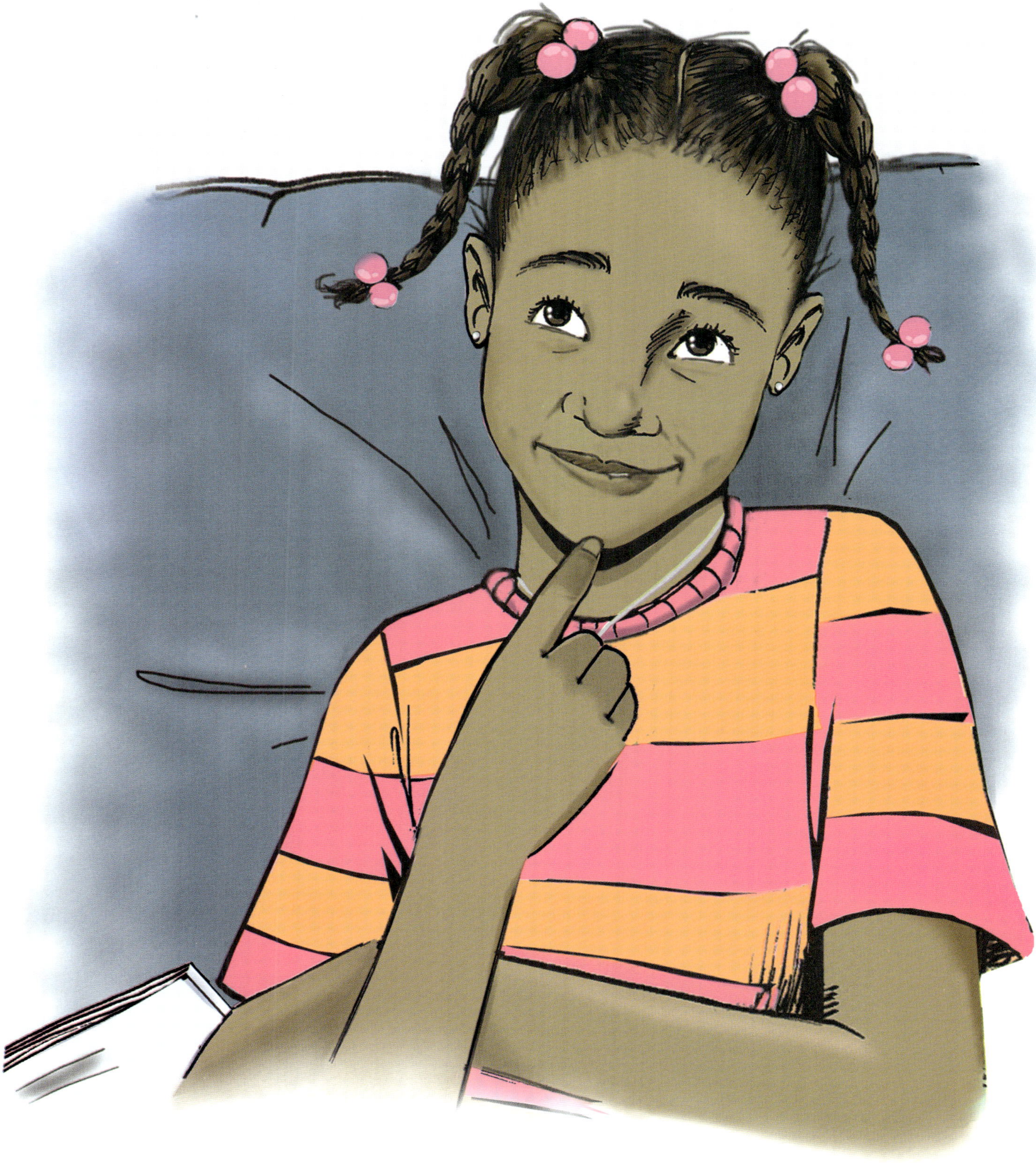

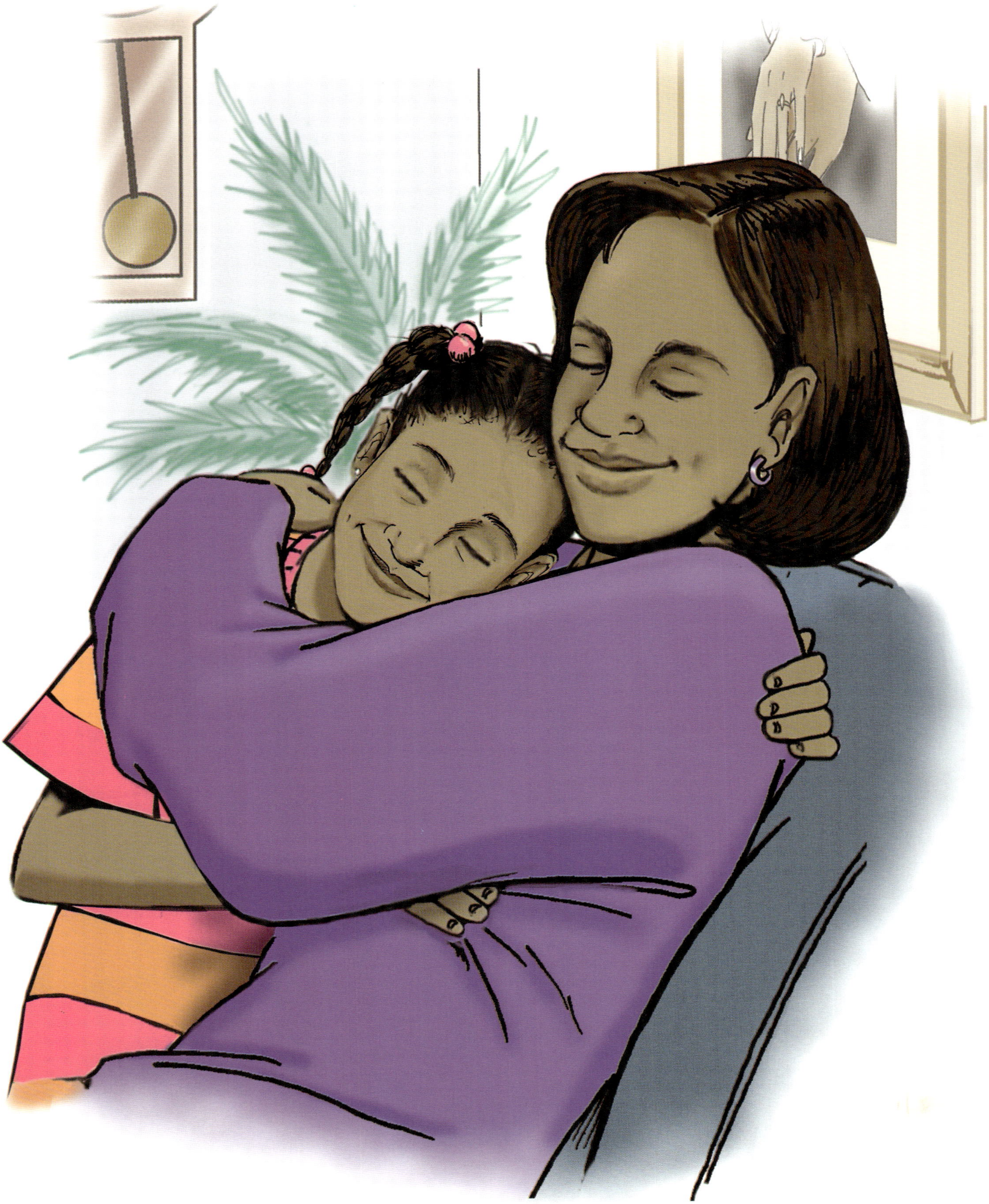

Regina brought the comb and brush. She gave them to her mother and asked, "Am I going to look pretty?"

"Sweetheart, you already look pretty!" She gave her daughter a big hug.

Her mother washed and conditioned her hair. Then she used a blow dryer. They went back into the family room. Regina sat down, and her mother parted her hair. Next, she brushed, combed, and began to style Regina's hair.

After twenty minutes, Regina asked, "Are you done yet?"

"No, sweetie. I'm not. Now turn your head and look down, please."

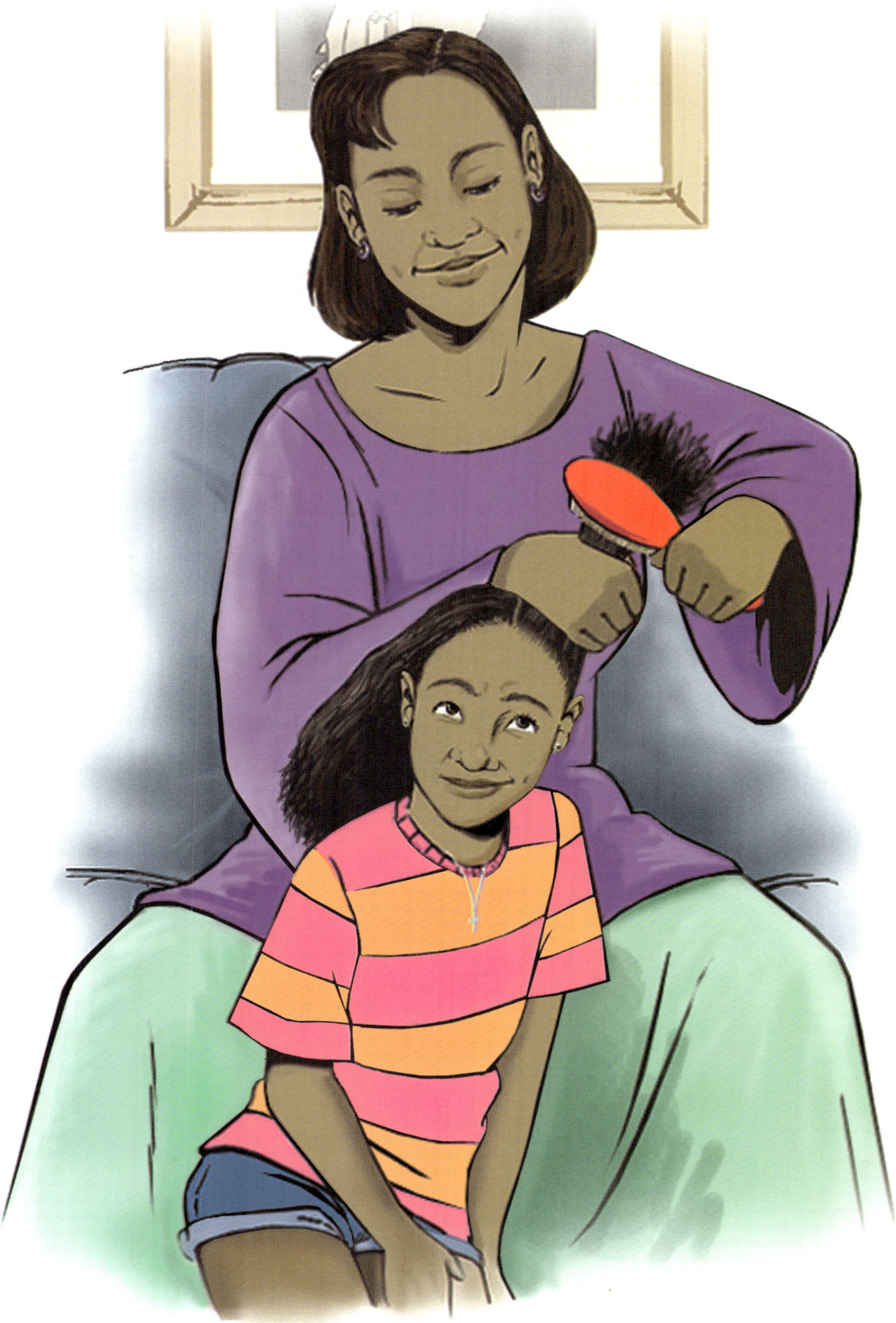

When her mother was finished, Regina jumped up, grabbed a book, and quickly asked, "Mom, can I go look in my mirror?"

"Sure," her mother answered, getting up and stretching.

When they got to Regina's bedroom, she looked in the mirror. She turned her head from left to right.

"Oh, Mom, you are the best braider in the world!"

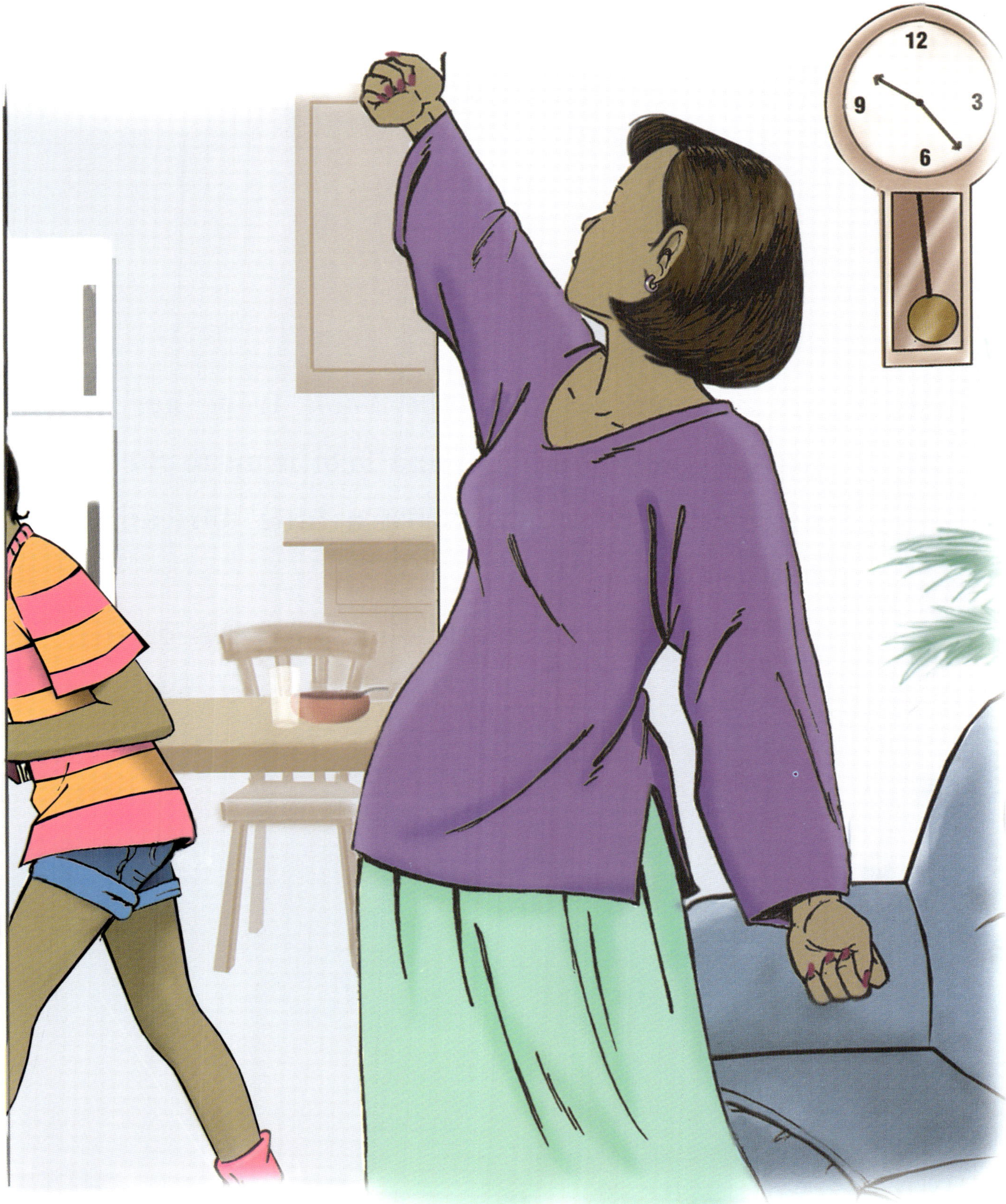
12
9
3
6

Her mother took the book from her, opened it to the middle, and held it up to the mirror. "Now you look like a little African Princess."

"No, Mom," said Regina. "An African Queen!"

They smiled.

◊ The name Regina (Latin) means "A queen."

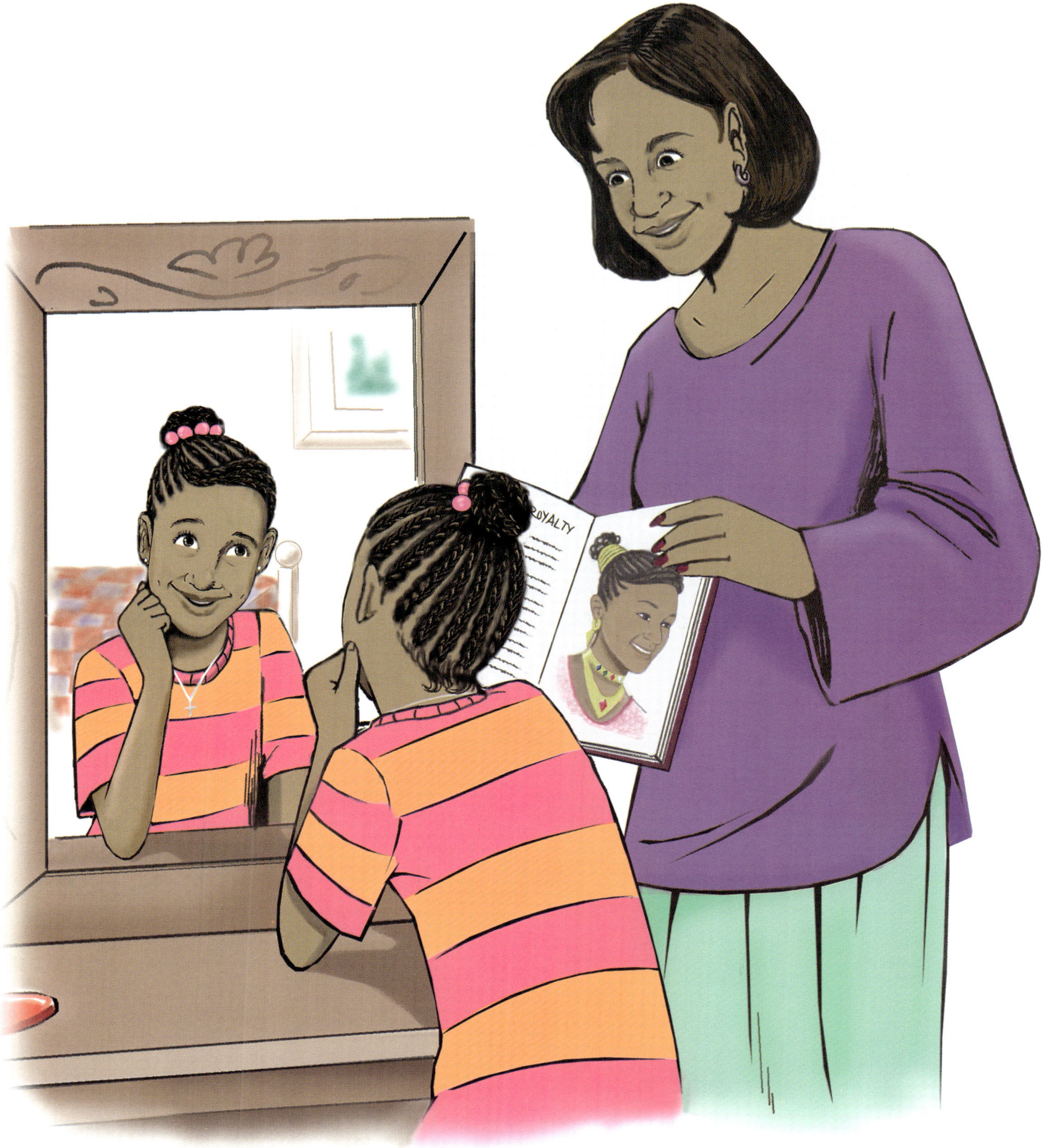
ROYALTY

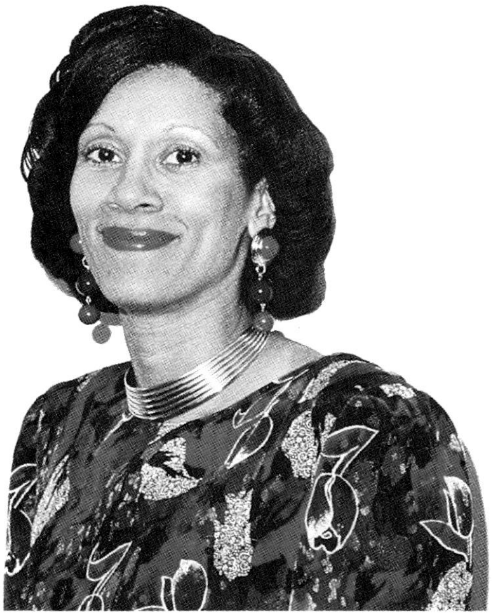

About the Author

Kathryn Diane Grace is happy about the many hairstyles available for young girls today. Being a military spouse, her family has moved nine times in 19 years. She found that young girls were the same everywhere. They were concerned about their appearance. Hearing the familiar phrase "A person's hair is their crown of beauty" led Mrs. Grace to write *Hairstyles for Me.* All of these hairstyles have been worn by her three daughters--Carrie, Carla, and Kristina.

Hairstyles for Me is Mrs. Grace's first picture book. She has also written two fiction novels for children, including *The Bike Hike* and *On With The Race!*

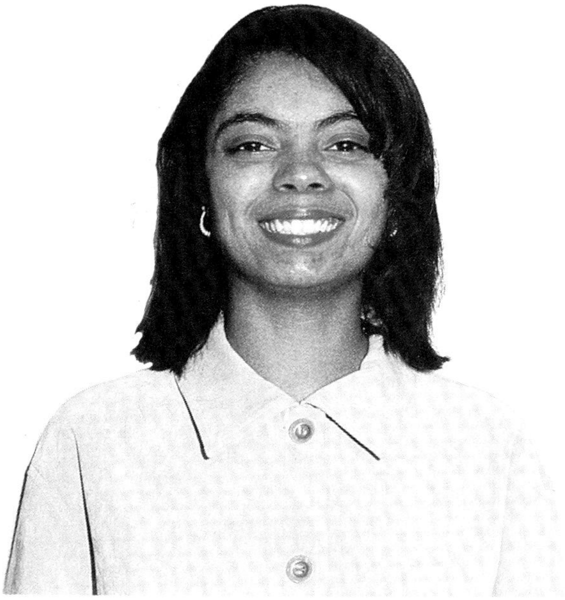

About the Illustrator

Aundrea Dionne Hernandez was blessed at an early age with the gift of drawing. She attended the San Antonio Art Institute and is working toward her Bachelor of Fine Arts.

Aundrea currently specializes in fine art and graphic design. This is her third published book. She currently lives in San Antonio, Texas, with her daughter, Kierstin.